Smart Diet

Healthy Raw food to keep you in shape for life

AMARPREET SINGH

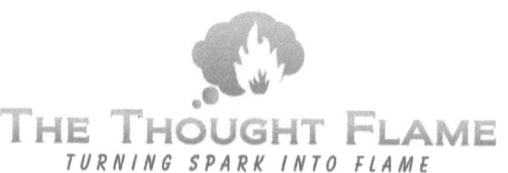

THE THOUGHT FLAME
TURNING SPARK INTO FLAME

info@thethoughtflame.com

www.thethoughtflame.com

Table of Contents

Introduction

Believe it or not raw food is extremely nutritious and rich in enzymes and energy. The point of the matter is that a raw food diet is simply one of the best diets ever. You would be surprised how popular this kind of diet is growing. The raw food diet is continuously gaining acceptance and respect throughout the world and is even become noticed in the mainstream medical community and it is about time.

While the rawfood diet is continuing to grow in popularity throughout the world, there are a number of books and other resources on the subject. Many of these resources that you will find contain many delicious recipes and helpful advice, but the truth is most of these resources are missing some crucial information: simple rawfood recipes.

Believe it or not rawfood recipes, while more complex than any traditional recipe, should take less time to make and should not be as complicated as many people believe they should be. Regardless of how hard you look, the truth is that you will not find a book that contains easy raw food recipes that are easy to make and take little to no time at all.

That is exactly what you will find in this eBook. This eBook is crammed filled with simple recipes that you can make and that follow any raw diet protocol. Most of the recipes that you will find greatly mimic many traditional cooked recipes that you love, but are completely healthy, leaving you feeling completely guilt free.

So, what are you waiting for? Let's get started making incredibly healthy rawfood diet recipes so that you can get the most out of your kitchen and get the chance to get out there and enjoy your life to its fullest.

Why Is A Raw Food Diet Beneficial?

It is no secret that when you begin a rawfood diet, you give your oven a break every once in a while. With this diet you are mostly eating healthy fruits, grains and vegetables, giving you almost little to no opportunity to use your oven.

The main idea behind this diet is that when you heat up food, it destroys most of the nutrients and natural enzymes that are put into the food. This is extremely bad for you as many of these important enzymes that is destroyed is used to help boost your digestive system and can even help you to fight off chronic diseases. To put it simply: when you cook it, you kill it.

Does It Even Work?

While it is true that you will most certainly lose weight on this diet, many raw foods are very low in calories, sodium and unhealthy fat. However, raw foods are high in fiber, which can help aid your digestive track.

While the rawfood diet has proven itself in numerous studies, there are a few things that you will need to be concerned about. For starters you will need to make sure that you are getting enough protein, calcium, iron and other important minerals and vitamins that you need as you will most likely not get them from your diet alone. This is because the raw food diet excludes anything that may come from an animal, so to ensure that you are getting everything that you need I highly recommend taking supplements while on the diet.

What Are You Not Allowed and Allowed To Eat While On The Diet?

There are different things that you will be allowed to eat while following this healthy diet such as:

Uncooked foods

Unprocessed foods

Organic foods

Fruits

Vegetables

Nuts

Various Seeds

Grains That Have Sprouted

Benefits of The Raw Food Diet

There are many benefits to following the raw food diet and that you will love most about it. Some of these benefits include:

1. Weight Loss

While weight loss is far from easy, there are different things that you can do to make it a bit easier. One way that you can make the process of losing weight easier on yourself is by following a raw food diet. When you eat raw food, it tends to take a longer time to digest, helping you to feel full for longer periods of time.

There are many different things that you can eat that would fit in the rawfood category such as:

Raw fish such as sushi and cured fish

Raw nuts and seeds

Raw cheese

Raw fruits and veggies

And much, much more...

2. Best For Your Overall Health

Many people do not understand exactly how good rawfood is for your overall health. Raw food can help detox your body as well as fully cleanse it, freeing your body of harmful chemicals, substances and bacteria. In fact there have been many people who have been able to cure themselves of chronic illness just by switching to a raw food diet. The point is that if you want to have a healthy life, then you should switch to a raw food diet, plain and simple.

3. Best Diet To Help Detox Your Body

If you are looking to rid your body of any harmful chemicals that could damage your body in the long run, the raw food diet is the perfect one for you. With the raw food diet, you are consuming the healthiest ingredients possible, all with components that are designed to detox your body such as important antioxidants, etc. If you want to cleanse your body, the raw food diet is perfect for you.

4. Incredibly Easy To Follow

There really is no other diet that is easier to follow than the raw food diet. While there are a couple of complicated recipes that you can make, I highly do not recommend doing so until you have been on this diet for a while. Making complicated recipes could frustrate you and deter you from your goal of living a healthier and happier life.

Now that you know some of the benefits of follow the raw food diet such as it can help detox your body or that it is incredibly easy to follow, the next thing that you have to do is begin making your own raw food diet recipes.

Tips To Starting An All Raw Food Diet

For those who have never gone raw before, it can seem pretty overwhelming at first. Regardless if you are trying out the diet for yourself for a week or for the rest of your life, there are a few things that you will need to do in order to start yourself off on the right foot. As with starting many new things, starting an all-raw diet will take some time to become accustomed to, but soon enough everything will be to become second nature to you.

In this section I will give you a few helpful tips that should help you on this new and exciting journey and will make the transition into an all raw food diet a little easier on you.

Tip #1: Stock Pile Your Pantry With All Of The Essentials

Before you can even begin diving into the world of raw food and preparing your very own meals, you will first need to make sure that you have all of the ingredients and supplies that you will need already on hand. I highly recommend getting some flax crackers to snack on throughout the day, cashews, plenty of fresh fruits and plenty of fresh vegetables. Remember, you can never have too many raw foods, as you will go through them fairly quickly anyway.

Tip #2: Educate Yourself As Much As Possible on The Topic of Raw Food

It is important that you understand the world of raw food and to become aware of it before starting this diet. Why is this? It will help you to better prepare yourself to answer some of the questions that you may already have pertaining to the subject. Also this will help you to educate others who may question your new diet choice so that you can give them the chance to understand exactly what it is that you are doing and why you are doing it.

Tip #3: Set Your Eyes On the Future

I always recommend to others that when it comes to planning a new diet and working towards the eng goal such as losing weight or becoming healthier, never worry about what you are doing right now. Always try to focus solely on the future and your future goals. Worrying about the present will only distract you. Focusing on the future will help to keep you motivated and will help to remind you why you are on this diet in the first place.

Tip #4: Plan Your Meals Beforehand

When starting any diet, the key to success is thorough planning. The same holds true for this kind of diet as thorough planning can help save you a lot of time and energy whether you are saving time shopping at the grocery store or saving energy preparing unnecessary meals. Always plan your meals ahead of time and always try to set up a scheduled meal plan weeks ahead of time. It will only help to make your life a lot easier.

Following these four simple tips can help you go a long way with this raw food diet. In order to be successful with it you will need to do a variety of things ranging from planning your meals ahead of time to educating yourself as much as possible on the subject. The more prepared you are to tackle on this lifestyle; the better it will be for your future.

<u>Raw Food Diet Soup Recipes</u>

Hearty Spinach Bisque

This is an incredibly hearty and creamy soup that you are going to absolutely love. Featuring just a touch of nutmeg and cumin, the fragrance of this recipe adds a warming and homey touch to it.

Ingredients:

1 Handful of Spinach, Organic, Fresh and Washed

1 Handful of Macadamia Nuts, Raw

2 to 3 Cups of Water, Warm

1 Tbsp. of Nutritional Yeast

1 Tbsp. of Miso

1 Clove of Garlic, Coarsely Chopped

1 tsp. of Cumin, Ground

½ tsp. of Chili Powder

½ tsp. of Nutmeg, Freshly Grated

Dash of Sea Salt and Pepper For Taste

Directions:

1. Place all of your ingredients into a blender and blend on the highest setting until completely smooth.

2. Pour into a serving bowl and season with a dash of nutritional yeast, salt, chili powder and pepper for taste. Serve at once and enjoy.

Savory Cream of Mushroom Soup

This is perhaps the most savory and flavorful soup that you will ever come across. Feel free to use whatever kind of mushrooms that you wish for this recipe or whatever kind of mushrooms are available in the super market at the time whether they are Portobello, White Button or Shitake.

Ingredients:

1 Handful of Mushrooms, Your Choice, Washed and Chopped Into Small Pieces

2 Cups of Water, Warm

1 Tbsp. of Butter, Hemp

1 Tbsp. of Miso

1 tsp. of Cumin, Ground

1 tsp. of Chipotle Powder

½ tsp. of Mesquite Powder

2 Sprigs of Thyme, Fresh

½ tsp. of Chili Powder

Directions:

1. Place all of your ingredients into a blender

and blend on the highest setting until completely smooth.

2. Adjust all of your seasonings for your personal taste.

3. Pour your soup into a serving bowl and garnish with some chili powder, sage and yeast. Enjoy.

Hearty Basil and Tomato Bisque

When it comes to utilizing your garden to its fullest, this recipe is the best one for you. I highly suggest using Heirloom tomatoes as they help to bring out the gorgeous color of this soup as well as bring this recipe a unique flavor that you are sure to love.

Ingredients:

1 Tbsp. of Amino Acids

2 Cups of Milk, Hemp

2 Heirloom Tomatoes, Large In Size, Seeded and Chopped Coarsely

1 Tbsp. of Flax Oil

1 Tbsp. of Honey, Raw

1 Handful of Basil, Fresh or Dried

Dash of Salt and Pepper For Taste

Directions:

1. Using a blender add in all of your ingredients and blend on the highest setting until smooth in consistency.

2. Season with a dash of salt and pepper for taste and serve at once.

Cucumber and Dill Soup

This is one of the best recipes to make on the days that you are feeling especially lazy. It utilizes fresh cucumbers and drill, which can be used straight from your own home garden. Whether you are making it to enjoy for yourself or are looking to impress a few guests, it is a great recipe to make.

Ingredients:

3 Cups of Water, Warm

2 Tbsp. of Hemp Seeds

2 Tbsp. of Dill, Fresh or Dried

2 Cucumbers, Large In Size, Peeled and Diced Finely

2 Tbsp. of Yeast, Nutritional

1 Tbsp. of Lemon Juice, Fresh

1 tsp. of Sea Salt

2 tsp. of Turmeric

½ tsp. of Thyme Leaves, Fresh or Dried

Directions:

1. Using a blender blend your cucumber first and blend until smooth. Remove from blender and add in your hemp seeds with water and blend until creamy in consistency.

2. Then add in the rest of your ingredients except for your dill and pepper and continue blending until smooth and creamy in consistency.

3. Pour your soup into serving bowls and garnish with a touch of black pepper and dill. Serve at once.

Traditional New England Corn Chowder

Whether you decide to use locally grown or organically grown corn, this recipe is sure to be one that you will thoroughly enjoy. This is a perfect dish to make during the summer months and it is one that nearly everybody in your family will fall in love with.

Ingredients:

1 Red Bell Pepper, Cored and Diced Finely

3 Ears of Corn, Fresh or Frozen

1 Stalk of Celery, Minced

½ of A Yellow Onion, Large in Size and Diced Finely

1 Tbsp. of Miso

1 Tbsp. of Chili Powder

1 tsp. of Kelp Powder

2 Cups of Water, Coconut

1 Tbsp. of Mesquite

1 Tbsp. of Honey, Raw

Dash of Sea Salt and Pepper For Taste

A Dash of Thyme Leaves, Fresh or Dried and Used For Garnish

Directions:

1. Place all of your ingredients into a blender except for your corn and garnish. Blend on the highest setting until smooth.

2. Next add in your corn and pour into a serving bowl. Garnish with your thyme and serve at once.

Raw Food Diet Appetizer Recipes

Fresh Seaweed Salad

You may be surprised to find that most sea vegetables are packed full of great nutrients and minerals that your body craves and needs. With this recipe you will be able to reap the rewards of using these great tasting ingredients while having a dish that is incredibly easy to make.

Ingredients:

½ Cup of Wakame Seaweed

2 Tbsp. of Honey, Raw

4 Tbsp. of Vinegar, Apple Cider

1 Tbsp. of Amino Acids

1 Clove of Garlic, Peeled and Minced

½ Cup of Carrots, Shredded

1 Handful of Scallions, Chopped

Touch of Flax Oil, Fresh

A Handful of Cilantro, Fresh and Minced

Dash of Red Pepper Flakes For Garnish

Dash of Sesame Seeds For Garnish

Dash of Sea Salt and Pepper For Taste

Directions:

1. Prepare your seaweed first by allowing it to soak in some water for a couple of minutes until it is soft and has expanded in size. Then drain and place into a medium sized bowl.

2. Add in the rest of your ingredients and toss gently until everything has been mixed together well.

3. Season with your sea salt and pepper and serve onto a plate. Add your garnish and enjoy immediately.

Delicious Tomato and Basil Delight

Sometimes the simplest dishes make the best dishes. This dish is one of them as it is both incredibly delicious and packed full of flavor that the whole family will enjoy. I highly recommend using heirloom or garden fresh tomatoes to get the best results.

Ingredients:

2 Tomatoes, Large In Size and Cut Into Thin Slices

1 Shallot, Medium In Size, Peeled and Minced

1 Handful of Basil Leaves, Fresh

1 Tbsp. of Vinegar, Apple Cider

Dash of Sea Salt and Pepper For Taste

Directions:

1. The first thing that you have to do is place one tomato slice on the edge of your serving plates. Continuing layering your tomato slices around the entire plate using a circular motion.

2. Sprinkle your fresh basil leave onto the plate along with your minced onion and shallots. Make sure you sprinkle both over your tomatoes.

3. Drizzle with your apple cider vinegar, sea salt and dash of pepper and serve immediately.

Filling Veggie Chips With Hummus

Whether you are looking to impress guests at a dinner party or whether you want to enjoy a healthy snack for yourself, this is one recipe that every person on a raw food diet must have in their cooking arsenal. By utilize "chips" made out of vegetables; this is a recipe free from grease and harmful additive, making it not only delicious, but incredibly healthy as well.

Ingredients:

½ Cup of Water, Warm

½ tsp. of Paprika, Ground

¼ Cup of Sesame Seeds, Grind In A Coffer Grinder Beforehand

1 tsp. of Sea Salt For Taste

½ Of A Zucchini, Medium In Size, Peeled and Chopped Finely

2 Tbsp. of Lemon Juice, Fresh

1 Tbsp. of Olive Oil

Directions:

1. Grind up your sesame seeds first until your make a fine powder. Set aside for garnish

2. Then place all of your ingredients into a small sized mixing bowl and mix together thoroughly until mixed well.

3. Serve into a serving dish and garnish with your powdered sesame seeds and serve with fresh cut vegetables of your choice and enjoy.

Tangy Flavored Jicama Salsa

This salsa is sweet, creamy and crunchy to the taste, making it one of the best salad/ salsa recipes that you will find anywhere. This is a dish you can make literally any time of the year, as it is great regardless of the season. Also it is incredibly easy to make, making the entire preparation process easier on you.

Ingredients:

1 Jicama, Peeled and Diced Finely

1 Clove of Garlic, Minced

1 Red Onion, Large In Size, Peeled and Chopped Finely

1 tsp. of Chili Powder

2 Avocados, Pitted and Sliced Into Halves

1 Tbsp. of Lime Juice, Fresh

1 tsp. of Cilantro, Fresh or Dried

Dash of Sea Salt for Taste

1 tsp. of Lemon Juice, Fresh

Directions:

1. Mix all of your ingredients together in a medium sized mixing boat, tossing gently to combine everything evenly.

2. Serve immediately and enjoy.

Creamy Cheesy Spread

This dish pairs perfectly with any other recipe that you imagining adding cheese to. Whatever your imagination can cook up, just go with it. I recommend making this in large batches and storing it in your fridge to use whenever you wish. This dish certainly goes great with a side salad or a plate of fresh veggies.

Ingredients:

2 Tbsp. of Yeast, Nutritional

1 Tbsp. of Butter, Hemp

1 Tbsp. of Lemon Juice, Fresh

1 Clove of Garlic, Peeled and Minced

1 Tbsp. of Mixed Herbs Such As Rosemary, Thyme, Basil and Oregano

½ tsp. of Turmeric, Ground

1 tsp. of Sea Salt For Taste

Directions:

1. Using a medium sized mixing bowl combine all of your ingredients together until mixed evenly. Add enough water to give it the consistency that you desire.

2. Store in a plastic container in your fridge and use whenever you are ready.

Raw Food Diet Entrée Recipes

"Nothing To It" Pasta

This is a pasta dish for pasta lovers without any of the guilt that goes along with it. The "noodles" that you will use are calorie free and contain all of the minerals that your body needs on a daily basis. Feel free to use different variation of the noodles until you are ready to come up with your own creative noodles.

Ingredients:

4 to 6 Tomatoes, Large In Size, Heirloom and Organic

1 Handful of Basil, Fresh and Torn

1 Yellow Onion, Medium In Size, Peeled and Diced Finely

½ Cup of Olive Oil

1 Clove of Garlic, Minced

1 Tbsp. of Red Pepper Flakes For Taste

1 tsp. of Chili Powder

¼ tsp. of Cayenne

1 tsp. of Honey, Raw

1 tsp. of Miso

Dash of Sea Salt For Taste

Directions:

1. Place all of your ingredients into a bowl and mash together using your bare hands.

2. Cover the bowl and set aside on your counter to sit for at least an hour.

3. Place veggie noodles of your choice on to a serving plate and top with your cover sauce. Serve at once and enjoy.

Homemade Raw BigMac

While you are on a raw food diet, you have probably never been prepared to enjoy a meaty hamburger again, did you? With this dish you will find yourself oddly satisfied as you mix most of the ingredients with your hands to create something almost meat-like. This is a great recipe to prepare if you are headed out to a barbeque or wish to change things up in your kitchen.

Ingredients:

2 Handfuls of Mushrooms, Diced Finely

4 Tbsp. of Yeast, Nutritional

1 Tbsp. of Shoyu

1 Tbsp. of Mesquite Powder

½ Of An Onion, Diced Finely

2 Carrots, Shredded

2 Tbsp. of Butter, Hemp Seed

1 tsp. of Vinegar, Apple Cider

1 Cup of Mixed Herbs Such as Coriander, Parsley, Thyme and Cilantro

Dash of Sea Salt and Pepper For Taste

Onions, Lettuce, Organic Mustard, Tomato and Ketchup For Toppings

Directions:

1. Using a large sized mixing bowl, combine all of your ingredients together until you have a thoroughly mixed and sticky mixture on your hands.

2. Then using your hands, form this mixture into patties. Serve as is and top with your favorite toppings. Enjoy.

Savory Layered Quiche

This is one of the most versatile and easiest recipes to prepare ever! Feel free to use whatever combination of vegetables and herbs that you want. You can serve this quiche during any time of the day and for the best results pair it with a fresh lunch salad.

Ingredients For Crust:

2 Cups of Coconut Flakes, Shredded

½ Cup of Water, Warm

½ Cup of Yeast, Nutritional

3 Tbsp. of Shoyu

1 Tbsp. of Miso

1 Tbsp. of Mesquite Powder

1 Tbsp. of Honey, Raw

¼ Cup of Basil, Dried or Fresh

Ingredients For Filling:

Meat From 1 Coconut, Young and Thai

2 tsp. of Turmeric

1 Tbsp. of Lemon Juice, Fresh

4 Tbsp. of Yeast, Nutritional

2 Tbsp. of Miso

2 Handfuls of Sprouts, Pitted and Finely Sliced

2 Handfuls of Dulse, Chopped

1 Handful of Raisins

2 Carrots, Diced Finely

1 Red Onion, Peeled and Sliced Into Small Circles

2 Tomatoes, Seeded, Heirloom and Finely Chopped

1 Handful of Arugula Leaves, Fresh

Directions:

1. Place all of your ingredients into a bowl and thoroughly mix until sticky.

2. Press your mixture into a pie plate and crimp the edges like you would with a pie. Place into your fridge until you are ready to fill it.

3. To prepare your filling use a blender to blend together your ingredients except for the arugula and tomato.

4. Once done blending pour your mixture into your crust. Cover your filling with your arugula leaves and tomato slice. Garnish with fresh basil and set in your fridge to chill until you are ready to serve.

Falafel With Sweet Corn

If you were a big fan of falafel you probably didn't realize that you could have it in a raw food form without worrying about cooking or adding beans to it. Even if you haven't heard of its raw form before, you do not worry that it will be dehydrated whatsoever. This dish is full of flavor and it is one that will leave you incredibly satisfied.

Ingredients:

4 Tbsp. of Butter, Hemp

1 Onion, Medium In Size and Minced

1 Cup of Coconut Flakes, Unsweetened

½ Cup of Cilantro Leaves, Fresh and Chopped Finely

½ tsp. of Cayenne Pepper

1 Tbsp. of Lemon Juice, Fresh

1 Tbsp. of Flax Oil

1 Tbsp. of Maca Powder

½ tsp. of Black Pepper For Taste

2 tsp. of Sea Salt

1 tsp. of Coriander, Ground

1 tsp. of Cumin, Ground

Directions:

1. Mix all of your ingredients in a medium sized bowl until thoroughly combined.

2. Then using your hands shape the mixture into small sized balls. Serve as is and enjoy.

Traditional Mac and Cheese

This is a perfect comfort dish without any of the guilt. It is incredibly easy to make the popular craft looking noodles just by using the sweet potatoes that this dish calls for and it will taste as close to the real thing as you can get.

Ingredients:

2 Sweet Potatoes, Large In Size, Peeled and

Sliced Into Thin Spirals

1 Clove of Garlic, Minced

½ Cup of Yeast, Nutritional

1 Tbsp. of Lemon Juice, Fresh

1 Tbsp. of Vinegar, Apple Cider

1 Tbsp. of Amino Acids

1 Tbsp. of Miso

Dash of Mustard, Stone Ground

½ tsp. of Chili Powder

¼ tsp. of Paprika

¼ tsp. of Turmeric

Dash of Thyme For Taste

Dash of Cayenne Pepper For Taste

1 Handful of Dulse, Shredded

Directions:

1. Mix all of your ingredients together in a small sized mixing bowl until the noodles are evenly coated.

2. Serve onto serving plates and enjoy at once.

Fettuccini With "Meatballs"

The sausage like meatballs that you make in this dish pair perfectly with the vegetable noodles that you are going to use. The great thing about this recipe is how versatile it is. Use the "meatballs" for this dish or make them slightly bigger to enjoy a "meatball" sub. Either way the choice is up to you. Spiced with a smoky flavor this recipe will surely not disappoint.

Ingredients To Make The Noodles:

2 Zucchini's, Peeled and Sliced Very Thinly To

Form Noodles

2 Sweet Potatoes, Peeled and Sliced Very Thinly To Form Noodles

Ingredients To Make The Sauce:

1 Clove of Garlic, Diced Finely

4 Tbsp. of Yeast, Nutritional

2 tsp. of Miso

Some Water To Make The Sauce Creamy

Dash of Sea Salt and Pepper For Taste

Ingredients For The Meatballs:

4 Tbsp. of Yeast, Nutritional

2 Tbsp. of Mesquite

1 Tbsp. of Maple Syrup

1 Tbsp. of Maca

1 Tbsp. of Butter, Hemp Seed

½ Of An Onion, Peeled and Diced Finely

½ tsp. of Cumin

½ tsp. of Pepper

½ tsp. of Nutmeg

½ tsp. of Oregano

½ tsp. of Marjoram

½ tsp. of Chipotle

½ tsp. of Paprika

1 Tbsp. of Basil, Dried

1 Tbsp. of Thyme, Dried

1 Tbsp. of Sage, Dried

Directions To Make The Sauce:

1. Mix all of your ingredients together in a medium sized mixing bowl until thoroughly combined. The sauce should have the appropriate consistency for sauce.

2. Once your "noodles" are sliced, pour the sauce over it and mix using your hands to ensure noodles are thoroughly covered.

Directions To Make The Meatballs:

1. Place all of your ingredients into a medium sized mixing bowl and mix thoroughly using your hands.

2. Once mixed use your hands to pack the mixture into small balls until your have a couple of "meatballs" in your hands. Add to your "fettuccini" and serve immediately. Enjoy.

Classic "Meatball" Sub

This recipe combines the perfect ingredients to make a meal that is hearty and completely satisfying to your taste buds. These "meatballs" go perfectly with a few cabbage leaves, tomatoes or even arugula leaves. Once you make this sandwich you will fall in love with it.

Ingredients:

1 Batch of Meatballs Used In The Last Recipe

A Few Leaves of Cabbage Leaves or Arugula

Ingredients To Make The Sauce:

1 Tbsp. of Olive Oil, Cold Pressed

2 Cloves of Garlic, Peeled and Minced

1 tsp. of Red Pepper Flakes

1 Handful of Parsley Leaves, Chopped Coarsely

1 tsp. of Oregano, Dried

2 Tomatoes, Heirloom, Seeded and Chopped Finely

1 tsp. of Sea Salt For Taste

1 tsp. of Black Pepper For Taste

1 tsp. of Honey, Raw

Directions:

1. Take your meatballs and place them into your cabbage leaves or arugula leaves.

2. Pour your marinara sauce over it to cover the meatballs. Garnish with some fresh basil and enjoy immediately.

Raw Food Diet Dessert Recipes

Spongy Layer Cake

While you are on the raw food diet, it can be hard to imagine that you can enjoy foods just like the rest of the world. This recipe not only looks amazing, but it tastes great and requires absolutely no baking. All that you need is a blender and that is it.

Ingredients For The "Cake"

2 Handfuls of Coconut Flakes, Unsweetened and Shredded

2 Tbsp. of Honey, raw

1 Tbsp. of Maca Powder

1 ½ Tbsp. of Butter, Hemp Seed

2 Tbsp. of Lucama Powder

3 Tbsp. of Coconut Oil

1 Tbsp. of Vanilla Extract

1 Tbsp. of Cinnamon, Powder

Ingredients For The Frosting:

Meat From 2 Coconuts, Young and Thai

1 Tbsp. of Vanilla Extract

1 Tbsp. of Cocoa Powder

1 Tbsp. of Lucama Powder

1 Tbsp. of Honey, Raw

1 Tbsp. of Coconut Oil

½ Cup of Water, Coconut

Ingredients For The Layer of Fruit

½ Cup of Strawberries, Fresh and Sliced

½ Cup of Cherries, DeSteemed and Diced

¼ Cup of Coconut Curls, To Be Used For Decoration

Directions For The "Cake"

1. Blend all of your ingredients together in a blender and blend until slight stiff in consistency.

2. Place in your fridge to allow for more stiffening.

Directions For Frosting:

1. Place all of your ingredients together in a blender and blend on the highest setting until smooth in consistency. Set aside.

Directions For Assembling Cake:

1. Using a spring pan, layer your cake first with the cake "batter", then the layer of fresh fruit, followed by another layer of cake batter and finishing off with your frosting.

2. Place your assembled cake into your freezer

to set and remove. Serve while frozen and enjoy.

Conclusion

There is nothing like starting a raw food diet. There are many benefits to doing so and it is an ideal diet to follow especially if you are looking to lead a healthier and much happier lifestyle. Whether you are looking to improve your health for a short time or simply for the rest of your life, you can do so with this diet.

With this eBook you have learned not only why a raw food diet is beneficial for you, but also some helpful tips to help you succeed with it and some great tasting raw food recipes. All of the recipes that can be found in this eBook are the simplest recipes that you will ever find, making them perfect for those just starting out on this diet. However, even if you have been on a raw food diet for some time now, I'm sure you would love to get a break from preparing complicated raw food recipes.

Now, the next thing for you to do is to begin making some of the recipes that you have discovered in this book. The best way to tell if you are going to enjoy this diet and reap the rewards from switching to this diet is to simply try it out for yourself.

About Us

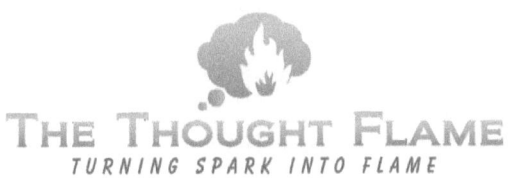

The Thought Flame is committed to add value to its customers through various books, online courses and other resources. You can learn more about us and our books at www.thethoughtflame.com.

Don't forget to check out our amazing **online video courses** at www.thethoughtflame.com/courses/ to take your knowledge to another level.

To check out our **extraordinary collection of diet/cookbooks**, visit http://www.thethoughtflame.com/category/non-fictional/cookbooks/ .

As a part of our valued relationship with our customers, we keep providing you free promotional books, courses and other stuff on subscribing with us on our site. We have a strict anti-spam policy and assure you no spam mails will be sent to your mailbox.

To subscribe with us, visit

www.thethoughtflame.com.

Like our work and would like to say thanks?

Buy us a cup of coffee at

www.thethoughtflame.com/coffee/

Author

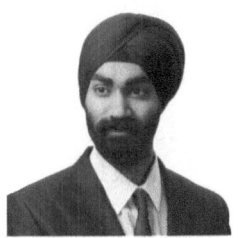

Amarpreet Singh is an avid learner and his passion for education has made him travel, work and study all across the world. He holds three masters degrees, including MBA, from top universities in Asia.

He is author of dozens of books, many of which are Amazon's bestseller, varying in various topics and categories. He also teaches many online courses having thousands of students across the world.

He has a keen interest in international affairs, economics, global poverty and politics, financial markets and entrepreneurship, and strives to be part of a community that shares the same passion.

He has worked as consultant with organizations like Airbus and The World Bank.

He loves travelling and learning about new cultures, and has been fortunate to live/work/travel/study in countries like India, China, Korea, US, South Africa, Japan, Philippines, Singapore, Canada etc., and learn about the culture and lifestyle in each of them.

To check out more of his work, visit www.thethoughtflame.com